S0-BLH-955

# Calcium and Nutrition

# Calcium and Nutrition

Laura Granger, MPH, RD

Publisher: Robert H. Garrison, Jr., MA, RPh

Editor In Chief: Elizabeth Somer, MA, RD

Managing Editor: Lisa M. Moye

Editorial Director: Janet L. Haley

Art Director: Scott Mayeda

Production Directors: Jeff Elkind, Irene Villa, Becky Moyer

Copy Editors: Norma Trost Foor, Jean Forsythe, Mary Houser,
Stephen C. Schneider, R. H. Garrison, Sr.

Cover Design: Stefanko & Hetz, Jeff Elkind

Photography: Bob and Irene Nishihira, Carlsbad, CA

Illustration: Jennifer Hewitson, Julian Naranjo, Walter Stuart

Copyright © 1986 by Health Media of America, Inc.

For information regarding volume purchase discounts contact:
Health Media of America, Inc.
11300 Sorrento Valley Road, Suite 250
San Diego, CA 92121

Printed in the United States of America.

ISBN 0-937325-08-2

# Contents

**Introduction**

# Introduction

Many Americans have realized that the familiar instruction from childhood, "Drink your milk," was possibly some of the best health advice they ever received. Calcium, a mineral found in milk and other low-fat dairy products, is linked with the prevention and treatment of numerous diseases including osteoporosis, high blood pressure (hypertension), cardiovascular disease, and cancer. Osteoporosis, an age-related disease that affects people age 45 years old or older, is responsible for 1.3 million fractures annually in the United States. One in every two deaths is a result of cardiovascular disease and 18% of adult Americans have hypertension, a major risk factor for stroke and heart attack.

Many questions remain for the consumer attempting to choose a diet and adopt a lifestyle that prevents these diseases. Many individuals want to know if they are at risk for developing a diet-related disease.

As Americans live longer, diseases such as osteoporosis that affect the older population are receiving increasing attention. Evidence suggests that there are ways an individual might be protected from developing osteoporosis and other degenerative diseases.

CALCIUM AND NUTRITION provides information on the functions of calcium, the best dietary and supplemental sources of the mineral, how much calcium is recommmended to prevent disease, why a calcium deficiency can cause osteoporosis or other disorders, and the possible effects of calcium overdose.

# 1
# Are Americans Getting Enough Calcium?

## How Much Calcium Do People Need?

The daily calcium requirement varies and depends on age, sex, and physiological state. The current Recommended Dietary Allowance (RDA) for adults is 800 mg of calcium daily. Children from 11 to 18 years old as well as pregnant or breastfeeding women need 1,200 mg per day. For infants up to a year old calcium needs are calculated based on body weight. An intake of 60 mg per kg (1 kg = 2.2 lb) of body weight is recommended.[1] This means that an infant weighing 6 kg (13 lb) should consume 360 mg of calcium daily, or the amount of calcium in 1 1/4 cups of milk. These recommended levels take into account that only about 30% of the calcium in foods will be absorbed by the body. *(Graph 1, Page 2)*

The RDAs are revised every few years as nutrition research provides new information. The adult RDA for calcium will probably increase to 1,000 mg when the RDA's are revised because of evidence that shows a daily intake of 800 mg might not be adequate to prevent or treat osteoporosis. The best intake to prevent degenerative diseases is not known. Some researchers suggest that 1,000 mg of calcium is not enough and that 1,500 mg of calcium is required to prevent age-related bone loss and osteoporosis.[2]

**Graph 1.** Calcium needs vary and depend on age, gender, and physiological state.

= 300 mg

**RDA Milligrams Needed Daily**

Children and Adults

= 800

Teenagers and Pregnant Women

= 1,200

Pregnant Teenagers

= 1,600

## The Calcium Content Of The American Diet

A low calcium diet is common in the United States. Several national nutrition surveys examined the adequacy of the diets of Americans and found them to be inadequate in calcium.[3,4]

In particular, women, older adults, and teenagers are at risk for calcium deficiency. Daily consumption of calcium is less than half of the RDA in those who do not drink milk.[5] *(Graph 2, Page 3)*

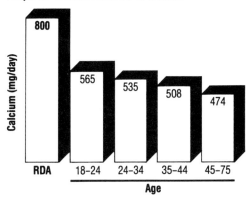

**Graph 2.   Calcium Intakes Of Women**

Males do better than females with an average estimated calcium intake of 700 mg/day. Intake is usually higher during adolescence and is lowest for men 50 years old or older. For females, the average intake is only 450 mg/day.[4] Dietary intake decreases with age; women 35 years old or older have the lowest intake of calcium.[6]

One in every two people consumes less than 100% of the RDA for calcium and over one-third of the population consumes less than 70% of the recommended 800 mg.[3] Intakes of less than 70% are cause for concern, especially with current evidence that suggests the recommendation of 800 mg might be too low to ensure prevention of osteoporosis.[2]

There are several reasons why Americans are not getting enough calcium.

**Reduced Consumption Of Low-Fat Dairy Foods:** Low-fat dairy foods, such as milk, yogurt, cheese, and cottage cheese provide three-quarters of the daily intake of calcium in the United States.[7] In contrast, fatty dairy foods, such as sour cream, cream cheese, cream, and butter supply little or no calcium. Limited intake of low-fat dairy foods might place a person at risk for calcium deficiency. Milk consumption has decreased in the United States and calcium is usually low in the diets of girls and women.[8] One of the causes for this reduction in calcium-rich milk might be soft drinks. Between 1960 and 1976, Americans reduced their annual intake of milk by five gallons each and increased soft drink consumption by 19 gallons a person.[9] The decrease in calcium and increase in phosphorus intakes that result from this dietary substitution might place a person at high risk for calcium deficiency.

**Lactose Intolerance:** Many people consume few dairy products because of an inability to digest these foods. Intolerance of dairy foods often stems from a deficiency of the enzyme, lactase. Lactase is needed for the body to digest the milk sugar called lactose. Without lactase, undigested sugar remains in the intestine and is consumed by bacteria that naturally inhabit this area. Symptoms such as gas, bloating, and diarrhea can result. A higher incidence of lactose intolerance is found in people with osteoporosis than in healthy people.[10] This finding supports the theory that inability to consume dairy products might be significant in causing osteoporosis.

**Weight Control Diets:** A diet that provides 1,600 calories or less might not supply adequate amounts of calcium. Many weight-watchers are women for whom an adequate calcium intake is important. Chronic dieters are a high risk group for calcium deficiency as well as marginal or low intakes of other nutrients.[3]

**Misconceptions About Calcium Needs:** Misinformation about calcium needs throughout life can result in inadequate intake of calcium. Many people think that calcium is necessary only during the growing years and that milk and high calcium intakes are not needed once bones are formed. This is not true. Bones are continually reformed throughout life. About 320 mg of calcium are excreted from the body every day, regardless of dietary intake. If the dietary intake of calcium does not replace the daily losses, a calcium deficit results and calcium is lost from the bone. Over time a chronic gradual loss of calcium can result in osteoporosis.

## Dietary Sources Of Calcium

Dairy products are the best sources of calcium. Low-fat milk and yogurt (35% of the calories come from fat) or nonfat milk and yogurt (less than .5% fat calories), and low-fat hard cheeses are the most concentrated sources of calcium. *(Figure 1, Page 6)* Ice cream, whole milk (50% fat calories), cottage cheese, and cheeses like cheddar or havarti provide calcium, but are high in fat. Non-dairy foods such as canned fish (with bones), oranges, tofu (soybean curd), and dark green leafy vegetables also contribute to calcium intake. Because of the oxalates in dark green leafy vegetables, these foods might not provide as much usable calcium as low-fat dairy sources. Oxalates are substances in foods that bind to calcium in the intestine and reduce its absorption.

An eight ounce glass of low-fat milk or yogurt, a two cup serving of cottage cheese, or a one and one-half ounce serving of low-fat hard cheese contains about 300 mg of calcium. To include at least 800 mg

**Figure 1. Dietary Contributors To Calcium Intake**

of calcium in the diet each day a person should consume at least two servings of milk, yogurt, or cheese. The additional calcium needs can be met by other foods in the diet. Those people who tolerate milk but prefer not to drink it might try the following techniques to increase their calcium intake.

- Add nonfat dry milk powder to casseroles, meatloaf, and cheese sauces. One tablespoon of nonfat dry milk supplies 52 mg of calcium and only 15 calories.
- Add nonfat dry milk to recipes for french toast, muffins, milkshakes, dips, puddings, pie fillings,

homemade breads and granola, and mashed potatoes (2 tablespoons to every one cup of potatoes).
- Add nonfat dry milk to creamy salad dressings.
- Cook rice and hot cereal in low-fat or nonfat milk.
- Use low-fat yogurt as a substitute for sour cream in recipes.
- Combine low-fat milk with nonfat dry milk solids and use instead of cream in soups and sauces.
- Use low-fat cheeses with fruit and crackers for snacks.
- Include several servings of calcium-rich vegetables in the daily diet.

People who cannot tolerate milk must plan their diets carefully to include an adequate amount of calcium. Meat, chicken, and fresh or frozen fish are poor sources of calcium. At least three servings each day must be included in the diet to ensure adequate intake. In addition, a person must receive frequent exposure to sunlight or a supplement of vitamin D to ensure calcium absorption.

Milk should not be eliminated from the diets of small children unless recommended by a physician. Children have small stomachs and a limited capacity for food. It is unlikely they can consume enough calcium on a diet without milk products because of the increased quantity of food that must be consumed. One good source of non-dairy calcium is fortified soy milk.

# 2
# Calcium:
# The Basics

**What Is Calcium?**

Calcium is a mineral found in abundance in the earth. It is one of the 22 minerals essential to the maintenance of the human body. Calcium, as well as phosphorus and magnesium, are classified as major minerals because they are found in large amounts in the body and the daily dietary requirements exceed 100 mg. In contrast, the trace minerals such as iron, selenium, and zinc are present in the body in smaller quantities and are required in the diet in amounts less than 20 mg a day. The terms "major" and "trace" do not reflect the degree of importance a mineral has in human health and nutrition; both categories of minerals are of equal importance.

Calcium is the most plentiful mineral in the body. Between 1.5% and 2% of an adult's weight comes from calcium, or between two to four pounds. Over 99% of the calcium in the body is found in bones and teeth where it combines in crystals with phosphorus, magnesium, fluoride, zinc, sodium, and other substances to form the rigid skeleton.[11] The skeleton provides support for the soft tissues of the body and holds the body erect. *(Figure 2, Page 10)*

A similar combination of calcium and other minerals is found in the enamel and dentin of teeth. Because the crystals are larger in the teeth than in the bone, the structure is harder and calcium does not move readily in and out of teeth as it does in bone.

9

**Figure 2.** Over 99% of the calcium in the body is found in the bones and teeth.

Even during calcium deficiency, little calcium is lost from the teeth. The remaining 1% of calcium in the body is found in the blood and other fluids of the body where it functions in blood clotting, transmission of nerve impulses, and activation of enzymes and hormones.

The bones serve as a large reservoir of calcium. Throughout the day, calcium is released from bones to be used for nerve transmission or muscle contraction and is absorbed from the blood into the bones when blood levels of the mineral are high, such as after a calcium-rich meal. *(Figure 3)*

During the growing years, the balance between calcium deposition and calcium removal from bone is weighted on the side of building and more calcium is deposited into bone than is removed. In the healthy adult, the balance between calcium in and calcium out is equal; about 600 mg to 700 mg of calcium enter and leave the bones each day.[12] In later years, especially if the diet is low in calcium or a person leads a sedentary life, more calcium is removed from the bone than is deposited.

The blood concentration of calcium must be maintained within a narrow range. The source of this blood calcium is the bones. Hormones, chemical messengers produced in body organs called endocrine glands, are important in maintaining the critical blood level of calcium. When blood levels are

Calcium passes out of the blood vessel and is absorbed into the bone.

Cross section of bone

Calcium is released from bone and enters the blood.

Capillary

**Figure 3. Bone Remodeling**
Calcium is released from bones and is absorbed from the blood into the bones.

low, hormones signal the bones to release calcium into the blood and blood levels increase. When blood levels of calcium are too high, hormones signal the bones to absorb the extra calcium and the blood levels return to normal. The amount of calcium obtained from the diet and the calcium excreted in the urine, stool, and perspiration or used to build new skeletal tissue also is important in calcium balance.

## What Does Calcium Do?

The formation and maintenance of bones and teeth are calcium's main functions. The other lesser known functions of calcium are also important.

## Blood Clotting

When the body is injured, calcium starts the healing process by stopping the bleeding with the formation of a blood clot. Normal blood calcium levels are maintained constantly to promote this process. Changes in the intake of dietary calcium will not have an effect on blood clotting.

## Membranes

Calcium is located in the membranes that surround all body cells. Calcium increases the stability of the membranes and helps regulate the flow of nutrients and other substances into and out of the cell.

## Muscle Contraction

Calcium, with the help of magnesium, regulates the contraction and relaxation of muscles. A person can lift a pencil, wash the car, or jog because of the relaxation and contraction of muscles that depend on an adequate amount of calcium. Muscle cramps can be associated with conditions that upset calcium levels in the blood. Calcium is an important contributor to the regulation of the heart beat because the heart is a muscle and the heart beat is a type of muscle contraction. Breathing also is a rhythmic muscle contraction and relaxation and requires calcium for its regulation.

## Nerve Transmission

Calcium is essential for transmission of nerve impulses from one nerve to the next. Without adequate calcium in the blood, the nerves become hypersensitive and send improper messages throughout the body. Tetany, intermittent and painful spasms of the muscles, can result. If blood levels of calcium are too high, nerve transmission is suppressed.

## Other Processes

Calcium assists in many important processes in the body. For example, the body's ability to use vitamin $B_{12}$ depends on an adequate concentration of calcium. Many enzymes also are dependent upon calcium. Enzymes work in the body by starting and speeding up chemical reactions. Calcium is essential for the enzymes that convert carbohydrates, proteins, and fats into energy for the body.

## Absorption Of Calcium

After a meal, complex digestive processes free the nutrients in the food for use by the body. The process of absorption refers to the transport of nutrients across the lining of the intestine into the blood stream or lymph. Once in the blood stream, nutrients can be used as is or converted to usable substances to perform their vital functions.

Calcium often occurs in combination with other substances in food. Calcium must be separated from these other substances before it is absorbed. This separation is most efficient in an acidic environment. For this reason, most of the absorption of calcium takes place in the upper three-quarters of the small intestine where the concentration of digestive acids is highest.

Humans are inefficient at absorbing calcium from the diet. Healthy adults absorb only 20% to 30% of the calcium ingested. Women who are past menopause absorb as little as 7% of their dietary calcium.[13] There are many factors that also influence calcium absorption. *(Table 1)*

## Factors That Increase Absorption Of Calcium

**Vitamin D:** Vitamin D is one of the most important factors in the absorption and use of calcium. Vita-

| Table 1 | Factors That Influence Calcium Absorption | |
|---|---|---|
| | **Increased Absorption** | **Decreased Absorption** |
| | Increased need for calcium | Alcohol |
| | Lactose (milk sugar) | Caffeine |
| | Vitamin D | Some medications |
| | Zinc (?) | High dietary phosphorus |
| | | High dietary protein |
| | | Excessive dietary fiber |
| | | Inactivity |
| | | Low vitamin D |

min D regulates calcium movement into and out of bone, and improves the body's ability to absorb calcium from the intestine. Vitamin D activates a carrier protein in the intestine that attaches to calcium. Once attached, calcium can cross the intestinal wall into the blood stream.[14,15] In addition to vitamin D from foods such as vitamin D-fortified milk, exposure to sunlight allows the body to manufacture its own vitamin D. When a person lives in overcast or smoggy areas or is not exposed to adequate amounts of sunlight, the diet becomes an even more important source of this vitamin.

Large doses of vitamin D might have the opposite effect of moderate intakes and could cause bone to lose its calcium and become weak.[16]

**Lactose:** Calcium absorption improves when lactose, the sugar found in milk and milk products, is also present. Milk is a good source of both lactose and calcium.[12] Lactose might impair the absorption of calcium in people who do not have sufficient amounts of the enzyme (lactase) to digest lactose. This condition is called lactose intolerance.

**High Calcium Need:** The body becomes more efficient at absorbing calcium when the need for the mineral is high. Pregnancy, lactation (breastfeeding), and the high rate of growth during childhood and adolescence are conditions that require more calcium.[12] During these stages the body may absorb up to 75% of the available calcium in the diet.[11]

**Zinc:** Adequate intake of zinc might be necessary for calcium absorption because evidence suggests that zinc influences the transportation of calcium across the intestinal lining into the blood.[17]

# Factors That Decrease Absorption Of Calcium

**Oxalates And Phytates:** Oxalates and phytates are substances found in some foods. They form complexes with calcium in the intestine and hinder absorption of the mineral.

Oxalates are found in rhubarb, chard, kale, spinach, cocoa, and soybeans. These foods also contain significant amounts of calcium. If a person eats a serving of spinach and also drinks a glass of milk, the oxalate might bind the calcium from the spinach but will leave the calcium from the milk free to be used.

Phytates are found in the outer husks of cereals such as oatmeal. People who regularly consume their calcium-rich foods at the same meal with high phytate foods might not benefit from the calcium source as well as if the calcium-rich food were consumed at a separate time from the phytate food. Phytates are destroyed if a whole grain is leavened with yeast and most breads or other grain foods that have added baker's yeast would not reduce calcium absorption.

**The Calcium And Phosphorus Balance:** Diets that contain about the same amount of calcium and phosphorus (a ratio of 1:1) improve calcium absorption. The average intake of phosphorus in the United States is between 800 and 960 mg daily; half of the population consumes more.[18] The ratio of calcium to phosphorus in the diet of most Americans is 1:2.8, almost three times the recommended ratio.[19] The high phosphorus-low calcium intake might be a result of a reduced consumption of low-fat dairy foods and an increased consumption of meat and phosphorus-containing soft drinks. *(Graph 3, Page 17)*

## Graph 3. The Calcium-Phosphorus Ratio Of Selected Foods

☐ Calcium  ■ Phosphorus

Liver, beef
8 mg
352 mg

Pork loin
12 mg
234 mg

Chicken breast
11 mg
214 mg

Frankfurter
32 mg
603 mg

Whole wheat flour
41 mg
372 mg

Lentils, mature seeds
79 mg
377 mg

Orange juice
11 mg
17 mg

Milk, cow's
118 mg
93 mg

Broccoli
103 mg
78 mg

Spinach, fresh
93 mg
51 mg

The calcium:phosphorus ratio has a greater effect on blood levels of calcium than the intake of calcium alone. Excess dietary intake of phosphorus or a poor intake of calcium in relation to phosphorus causes the body to excrete calcium in the urine and increases calcium loss from bones.[11,19]

**Protein Intake:** A high-protein diet increases the excretion of calcium in the urine and the dietary requirement for calcium must be increased to compensate for the loss.[4,20] The American diet is high in protein. People often consume two to three times the RDA for protein and this dietary habit, coupled with low calcium and high phosphorus intake, increases the risk for calcium deficiency.

**Low Vitamin D Intake:** Calcium deficiency and bone disorders can develop in spite of adequate calcium intake if the diet is low in vitamin D. This fat-soluble vitamin is required for calcium to be absorbed and used in the body.

**High Fiber Intake:** The fiber in whole grain breads and cereals might bind to calcium in the intestine and reduce its absorption. The total fiber intake from a diet of whole grain breads and cereals, fresh fruits and vegetables, low-fat dairy products and meats probably will have little effect on calcium absorption. However, if a person consumes large amounts of processed fiber such as bran, and consumes a diet marginal to low in calcium, a calcium deficiency might result.

**Alcohol And Drugs:** Factors other than diet can also affect the body's use of calcium. While moderate alcohol consumption appears to have no effect, alcoholics absorb calcium less efficiently and might develop abnormal bones.[20] Use of certain drugs such as tetracycline, thyroid preparations, diuretics, and aluminum-containing antacids also can decrease absorption of calcium.[13]

**Other Lifestyle Factors:** Individuals who are bedridden or inactive might absorb less calcium and lose more calcium from the bones.[21] Stress also is associated with an increased loss of calcium and a higher intake of the mineral might be required during stressful times to maintain normal calcium balance.[11,12]

# 3
# Calcium And Osteoporosis

It is difficult to pick up a newspaper or magazine today without reading about the bone disease osteoporosis. Scientists are trying to determine all the causes of osteoporosis, who is at greatest risk for developing this disease, and what steps might be taken to prevent or cure it.

## What Is Osteoporosis?

Osteoporosis is the most common bone disease in the world; one in every four women will develop osteoporosis and 15 million people currently have it.[22,23] It is caused by chronic loss of calcium from the bones and is characterized by pain and crippling caused by weak, porous, bones that break easily. Bone loss is a result of aging and is most commonly seen in advancing years in both men and women. However, the rate of bone loss varies among individuals and with the type of bone affected. Fractures of the hip, wrist, and vertebra (backbone) are common.[24]

## Bone Structure

Bone is comprised of a tough framework of protein that is strengthened by deposits of calcium. Mature bone is about 30% protein framework and 70% mineral deposits. The newly formed bones of small children have a higher percentage of framework to mineral content.

The framework of bone is mostly strands of protein fibers, called collagen, that criss-cross to form a web. This gives bones the flexibility to withstand pressure without cracking.

The spaces within this protein framework are filled with crystals composed primarily of two minerals, calcium and phosphorus. Other minerals, such as magnesium, fluoride, zinc, and sodium also are found in the framework.[25] These minerals give strength and rigidity to the bone tissue. The more tightly packed the minerals and the larger the crystals that form in bone, the denser and stronger the bone tissue. *(Figure 4, Page 22)*

The protein framework gives bone its strong tensile strength, or ability to withstand tension. The mineral crystals are similar to marble and allow bone to resist compression and withstand the weight of the body and physical activity. This ability of bone to withstand pressure and compression is similar to the qualities of reinforced concrete. The steel rods of reinforced concrete provide the flexibility and tensile strength and the cement gives the structure compression strength. Healthy bone, however, is stronger than the finest reinforced concrete.[25]

Bone undergoes continual remodeling throughout life; existing bone minerals are removed and are replaced with new minerals. These processes are known as bone deposition (adding calcium to bone) and bone resorption (removing calcium from bone). Bones reach a maximal strength and density when an individual is 35 years old. After reaching this peak, strength and density continue to decline for the remainder of life, a result of greater bone resorption than deposition.

**Figure 4.** Mature bone is composed of mineral crystals embedded in a protein framework.

Bone mass is a measure of the strength or density of the bone. Men have a bone mass 25% to 30% higher than women, so men's bones are more dense. Black people have a 10% higher bone mass than white people, which might explain the reduced incidence of osteoporosis in this population.[26] Reduction of bone mass over time results in weak bones that are more brittle. It is the reduction of bone mass that is a primary cause of the broken bones or fractures seen in osteoporosis.

There are actually two types of bone loss that occur throughout life. The first involves a bone tissue known as cortical or compact bone. This type of bone tissue is found in the long arm and leg bones. Loss of cortical bone escalates after an individual is 50 years old and is often experienced by women after menopause.[16]

The second type of bone loss affects the bones in the spine and pelvis. These bones are called trabecular bones. They are less compact than cortical bone and have a honeycomb-like appearance. As early as the third decade of life both men and women begin to steadily lose trabecular bone.[16]

## What Are The Symptoms Of Osteoporosis?

For some individuals the first symptom of osteoporosis is a bone fracture. Other individuals may suffer from years of other aches and pain often attributed to "getting older." Research suggests that bone loss might occur first in the jaw bone, followed by the ribs and vertebrae (bones of the spine).[27] Loss of calcium from the jaw bone, with accompanying pain, could cause further problems by increasing the chances of losing teeth, which would limit the variety of foods and calcium in the diet.

Women suffer from fractures of the spine more often than men.[26] These fractures are known as compression fractures because the vertebrae of the spine are compressed together. Routine activities such as lifting an object or rising from a chair can cause a bone in the spine to collapse if a person has osteoporosis. This type of fracture does not always cause pain and a person may not know it has occurred. It is the repeated collapse of vertebra that is responsible for the loss of body height (up to 8 inches) and curving of the spine (dowager's hump) that is observed with aging.[28] *(Figure 5, Page 24)*

Another common fracture seen in osteoporosis is the hip fracture. It is estimated that 190,000 hip frac-

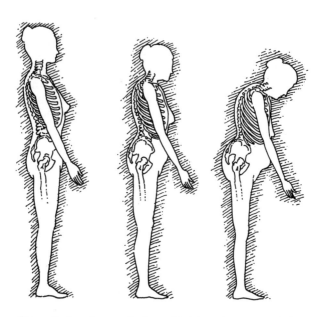

**Figure 5.** In osteoporosis, loss of height and curvature of the spine are caused by calcium loss from the bones.

tures occur each year and two-thirds of these are caused by osteoporosis. By age 90, 33% of women and 17% of men have suffered hip fractures.[21,22] Complications such as hospitalization, depression, and surgical problems often accompany hip fractures. These complications prove fatal for 12% to 15% of the sufferers, placing hip fractures as the second leading cause of death among people 47 to 74 years old.[22]

The extent of damage from osteoporosis is greater than a loss in height, pain, dental disease, and fractures. Those who survive the hip fracture often lose their mobility and independence and must rely on family, neighbors, or nursing home staff. The depression or fear of future falls that can accompany the disease reduces the quality of a person's life. The loss of teeth that results from deterioration of the jaw bone can cause eating disorders and malnutrition, which further reduces a person's resistance to disease and infection.

The long-term and serious effects of osteoporosis emphasize the importance of prevention and effective treatment of osteoporosis.

## Who Is At Risk For Developing Osteoporosis?

All people are at risk for developing osteoporosis since bone mass declines with age. However, factors in a person's genetic background and lifestyle can influence the rate of development and extent of damage.

**Women:** Women are eight times more likely than men to develop osteoporosis. Women's bones are thinner and less dense than men's bones, and less calcium must be lost before the bones are too weak to support the weight of the body. Women tend to live longer than men and because osteoporosis is linked to the aging process, women are at greater risk for the disease. In addition, women consume less food than men and are more likely to be on weight loss diets that restrict food, and calcium, intake.

White women with a northwestern European ethnic heritage appear to be at greatest risk for developing osteoporosis. These women often have fair complexions with freckles and blond hair. Women of Mediterranean descent have a lower incidence of osteoporosis. Black women seldom suffer from this bone disorder. Osteoporosis is also more common in lean women than in obese women.[29]

**Heredity:** If a person has inherited a small, thin skeleton, he or she has less calcium to lose before the bones are unable to support the weight of the body. Calcium intake and exercise throughout life are important for these people.

**Menopause:** Bone mass decreases at a faster rate after menopause. This decline in bone mass after menopause is attributed to a decrease in the blood level of estrogen, a female hormone produced by the ovaries, and to chronic low intake of calcium throughout life. When estrogen decreases, bone tissue becomes more sensitive to the hormone, which signals calcium to leave the bone.[22] As a result, the process of bone loss increases after menopause. Women who have an early menopause brought about by surgical removal of the ovaries are at high risk for developing osteoporosis.[26]

It is a mistake to think, however, that osteoporosis begins in later life. Any signs of bone loss at this stage are an indication that the process of calcium depletion has been progressing for years and becomes apparent or is accelerated after menopause.

**Low-Calorie Diets:** Consumption of a low-calorie diet promotes osteoporosis.

A woman who consumes a low-calorie diet is at risk for developing osteoporosis because a low-calorie diet is often a low-calcium diet. If a woman diets throughout life the likelihood of chronic low intake of calcium increases. A diet of less than 1,600 calories might not supply adequate calcium and supplementation should be considered. Half of the women in the United States consume less than 1,493 calories a day and are at risk for several nutrient deficiencies, including calcium.[1,4]

A reliance on regular or diet soft drinks that contain phosphorus can upset the ratio of calcium to phosphorus and increase calcium loss from bones.

**Sedentary Lifestyle:** Exercise increases bone mass and reduces bone loss.[26,30] Without physical activity, the bones rapidly lose minerals. The type of exercise most helpful in the prevention of osteoporosis is exercise that puts weight and stress on the long bones of the body. Examples of weightbearing exercise are walking or jogging.

The most dramatic example of the effects of lack of physical activity on bone health can be drawn from the experience of early astronauts. After 72 hours in the weightlessness of space, a group of young astronauts lost significant amounts of calcium from their bones.[31] The effect of weightbearing on bone strength may also explain why slender women are more prone to developing the disorder than their obese counterparts whose skeletons support more pounds.

**Stress:** The body absorbs less calcium during times of stress, tension, and grief. Stress should be minimized or calcium intake should be increased to compensate for the reduction in absorption.

**Pregnancy:** At one time it was thought that pregnancy and lactation (breastfeeding) drained calcium from the body and a woman's skeleton would be weakened by her developing baby. More recently it has been observed that women with a history of two or more pregnancies actually have a lower risk for osteoporosis. The preventive effect of pregnancy on osteoporosis might result from the effects of increased weightbearing during the pregnancy.

**Medications:** Individuals who require long-term use of certain medications also might need calcium supplementation. Corticosteroids can interfere with calcium absorption. The antibiotic tetracycline forms a complex with calcium that interferes with both absorption of calcium and the medication.[32]

Certain types of diuretics (water pills) may cause an increased loss of calcium in the urine. Isoniziad, a drug used in the treatment of tuberculosis, can depress calcium absorption.[33] Over-the-counter antacids that contain aluminum can also cause problems. *(Table 2)*

The possible interactions of drugs and nutrients can be serious and are often overlooked. Individuals who take the below medications should consult their physicians before adding any supplements or over-the-counter medications to their health care program.

**Coffee Drinkers:** Caffeine increases the amount of calcium excreted in the urine.[21] High intakes of caffeine beverages (6 or more cups of coffee daily) might lead to a negative calcium balance where more calcium is lost from the system than is replaced.

| Table 2 | Medications That Affect Calcium |
|---------|--------------------------------|
| 1. | Corticosteroids (anti-inflammatory) |
| 2. | Diphenylhydantoin (anticonvulsant) |
| 3. | Diphosphonates (Paget's disease) |
| 4. | Furosemide (diuretic) |
| 5. | Glutethimide (sedative) |
| 6. | Isoniazid (tuberculosis) |
| 7. | Phenobarbitol (anticonvulsant) |
| 8. | Primidone (anticonvulsant) |

While the best plan is to be moderate in caffeine consumption, those unwilling to lower their intake might need to consider use of a calcium supplement.

**Cigarettes And Alcohol:** Cigarette smoking and a heavy intake of alcohol are other habits associated with the development of osteoporosis.[11,26]

## Diagnosis Of Osteoporosis

The lack of simple, objective tests to measure bone loss has made the study of osteoporosis difficult. There is no blood or urine test that can diagnose osteoporosis. There are several methods available to measure bone density. These techniques vary in their cost, availability, and, since they rely on X-rays, radiation dosage. In addition, as much as 30% of bone must be lost before a standard X-ray will detect the presence of osteoporosis.[29]

Bone depletion can first be detected in the bone of the jaw, called the alveolar bone. This depletion of bone tissue occurs much earlier than osteoporosis and is associated with a reduced intake of calcium. If bone loss is detected at this point, the process might be reversed by increasing the consumption of calcium to at least the recommended level of 800 mg daily.

A method of detecting the early stages of osteoporosis is called Radiographic Densitometry. It uses common dental office X-ray equipment and allows evaluation of bone status during a person's routine dental examination.[27]

## Prevention Of Osteoporosis

The pain and suffering caused by osteoporosis might be prevented. While treatment of osteoporosis is possible, the best defense is prevention.

Prevention begins early. If a person is between 20 and 40 years old, he or she has reached adult height. Bones have reached maximum length and width and unless careful attention is paid to diet and exercise, bones will begin to lose calcium.

If a person is more than 40 years old, the bones have begun their thinning process. Although this is a normal process, if it proceeds too quickly or lasts for a long time, the possibility of osteoporosis increases. The rate of bone loss can be slowed if calcium intake is increased and "weightbearing" exercise is a part of the daily routine.

The following steps will help prevent this disease:

1. Consume adequate calcium (800 mg to 1,200 mg) and vitamin D (400IU) throughout adult life. After menopause, women who are not receiving estrogen therapy should consume about 1,500 mg of calcium per day.[26]
2. Engage in weightbearing exercise such as walking or jogging on a daily basis.
3. Avoid cigarette smoking. Women who smoke reach menopause several years earlier than non-smokers and are at increased risk for developing osteoporosis.[16]
4. Do not take large doses of vitamins A and D. Excesses of these vitamins will cause the body to lose strengthening minerals from the bones.[16] *(Figure 6, Page 31)*

## Treatment Of Osteoporosis

Treatment of osteoporosis is similar to the recommendations for prevention. Early detection is essen-

**Figure 6. Foods High In Calcium**

1. **Milk Group**
   Nonfat milk
   Yogurt, plain
   Swiss cheese

2. **Fruit-Vegetable Group**
   Bokchoy
   Mustard greens
   Turnip greens

3. **Grain Group**
   Cornbread

4. **Dried Beans And Meat Group**
   Beans, dried, cooked
   Salmon, with bones
   Sardines, with bones
   Tofu, processed with
      calcium sulfate

tial to begin treatment of osteoporosis before a disabling fracture occurs.

**Estrogen Replacement:** Estrogen levels decline at menopause. For women entering menopause, one of the most effective forms of treatment for osteoporosis might be estrogen replacement therapy. Women who receive estrogen replacement therapy within a few years of menopause have fewer hip and wrist fractures than those who do not receive treatment.[26]

Estrogen replacement therapy, however, might increase the risk for some types of cancer such as cancers of the uterine lining. Estrogen replacement therapy might not be appropriate for all women.[34]

**Calcium And Vitamin D Supplements:** Supplements that combine both calcium and vitamin D are another common treatment for osteoporosis. Individuals need more vitamin D as they get older. People in northern climates or older people who are not exposed to enough sunlight may have difficulty meeting their vitamin D requirement. In addition, older adults might not produce as much vitamin D in the skin, even when they are in the sun, as they did in former years.[35] As a result, adding a moderate amount of vitamin D to a calcium supplement might make the treatment more effective. To avoid possible toxic effects, no one should consume more than 600 to 800IU of vitamin D daily.[26]

**Fluoride:** People who grow to adulthood in areas with a high fluoride level in the water have a lower incidence of osteoporosis than those who are in a low fluoride area.[36] Fluoride is effective in increasing the bone mass in the spine and hip. One major side effect of fluoride is gastrointestinal irritation. It is still too soon to say who fluoride might help and how to determine the ideal dosage.[16]

## Can Osteoporosis Be Reversed?

There is evidence that some of the bone loss of osteoporosis might be reversed if discovered early and promptly treated. One study used calcium and vitamin D supplementation in a group of elderly women age 79 to 89 years old. After three years of consuming an intake of over 1,000 mg calcium per day, these women had a bone density 12% higher than similar women who consumed an average of 450 mg of calcium per day.[27]

In another experiment, healthy women 37 to 73 years old were given 750 mg of calcium combined with 375 IU of vitamin D. After 36 months on this regimen, the women showed an average increase in bone density of 12.5%.[37]

The density of the jaw bones in a group of people was increased by giving each of them 1,000 mg of calcium daily for 12 months.[38] Jaw bone strength and tooth disorders are improved when calcium intake is increased.[39]

Exercise also has been used to increase bone density. In a group of 73 postmenopausal women, those who participated in exercises of walking or dancing increased their bone strength. A similar group of women who did not exercise continued to lose bone mass.[30] Results of these studies offer hope for those who are already experiencing some of the debilitating symptoms of osteoporosis.

People who want to reduce their risk for osteoporosis should consume a diet adequate in calcium and vitamin D, avoid cigarette smoking and use of excessive vitamin D or vitamin A supplements, and engage in regular weightbearing exercise. Currently treatment for osteoporosis relies on estrogen replacement therapy and supplementation with calcium and vitamin D.

# 4
# Calcium And Hypertension

Blood pressure is the pumping force of the heart as it sends blood through the arteries to all tissues of the body. Each time the heart beats, the blood pressure increases momentarily. This is called systolic blood pressure. Between beats, the heart relaxes as it refills with blood. The residual pressure in the arteries between beats is called diastolic blood pressure.

Blood pressure is measured by placing a rubber cuff around the upper arm and inflating the cuff with air. This inflated cuff presses against the artery and closes it off. As the air is released gradually from the cuff, the blood begins to flow again through the artery and the pressure at which it flows is recorded on a measuring gauge or digital read-out.

More than 60 million people in the United States have high blood pressure (hypertension).[40] Hypertension is excessive pressure of the blood against the walls of the heart and arteries. Hypertension is diagnosed when a person has a blood pressure reading that averages 160/95 or more on two or more successive occasions. Blood pressure varies during the day and from one day to another. Hypertension occurs when the blood pressure remains elevated.

## Blood Pressure Values

|  | Systolic/Diastolic |
| --- | --- |
| Normal . . . . . . . . . . . . . . . . . . . . . . | 120/80 or less |
| Borderline . . . . . . . . . . . . . . . . . . . | 140/90 to 160/95 |
| Hypertension . . . . . . . . . . . . . . . . . . | 160/95 or more |

Blood pressure is regulated by a thin layer of muscle that surrounds the artery walls. The muscle can expand (relax) to increase the diameter of the artery and allow more blood to move through with less pressure when blood pressure is too high. The muscle can constrict (contract) to reduce the diameter of the artery and increase blood pressure when the pressure falls too low.

Hypertension occurs when muscles of the arteries contract and stay contracted, when blood volume increases, or when the heart's pumping action increases. Regardless of the origin, hypertension is a result of either an increased blood volume or reduced diameter of the arteries. *(Graph 4, Page 36)*

For 90% of people with high blood pressure there is no known cause. This type of hypertension is called "essential hypertension." The remaining 10% have hypertension that can be attributed to another disease such as a tumor on the adrenal gland or diabetes.[41] This type of hypertension is called "secondary hypertension."

Many factors influence an individual's blood pressure: age, race, heredity, body weight and percent body fat, stress, cigarette smoking, oral contraceptives, pregnancy, exercise, and nutrition. Certain medications including oral contraceptives, steroids, nasal decongestants, appetite suppressants, and some types of antidepressants also might cause secondary hypertension in some people.[40] In the United

**Graph 4.** Hypertension occurs when muscles of the arteries contract, when blood volume increases, or when the heart's pumping action increases.

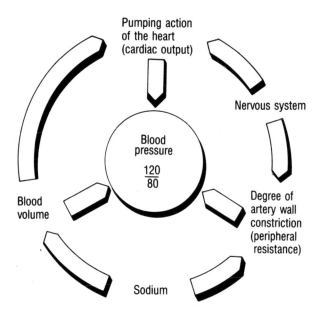

Pumping action of the heart (cardiac output)

Nervous system

Blood pressure

120
80

Blood volume

Degree of artery wall constriction (peripheral resistance)

Sodium

States, blood pressure tends to increase in individuals with age. Hypertension is more common and occurs at an earlier age among blacks.[42]

Hypertension has earned the label of the "silent killer" because those who have it often do not have symptoms and might not seek the necessary medical care. Two in every five people who have hypertension do not know they have it.[43] Feelings of stress, increased heart beat, or being "uptight" are not symptoms of hypertension. The only way to detect hypertension is to have regular blood pressure checks.

Hypertension is dangerous because it accelerates the process of atherosclerosis and heart disease. People with hypertension have a two to three times greater chance of developing heart disease, and a three times greater chance of having a stroke than people with normal blood pressure. People with hypertension have an increased risk for developing blood clots that can block an already cholesterol-clogged artery and cut off blood supply to the heart or brain.[43] Elevated blood pressure weakens the arteries and encourages them to break (aneurism). Although hypertension (high blood pressure) is a major risk factor for developing cardiovascular disease (CVD), congestive heart failure, stroke, and chronic kidney failure, the risks of disability or death from hypertension can be reduced with proper treatment. *(Figure 7, Page 38)*

## Nutrition And Hypertension

Nutrition is important in the cause, prevention, and treatment of hypertension. In the past, studies relating nutrition and hypertension focused on sodium. Sodium is a mineral found in table salt. Sodium also is used as a food additive, such as monosodium glutamate (MSG) and the sodium nitrite in processed meats.

Studies that compare large population groups throughout the world show that the higher the salt intake of the people in a country, the higher the blood pressure of its people.[44] In areas of South Africa and New Guinea where sodium intake is very low (200 to 1,400 mg daily), hypertension is almost absent. High blood pressure is prevalent in northern Japan, where the intake of sodium often exceeds 9,200 mg per day.[45]

**Hypertension: Target areas**

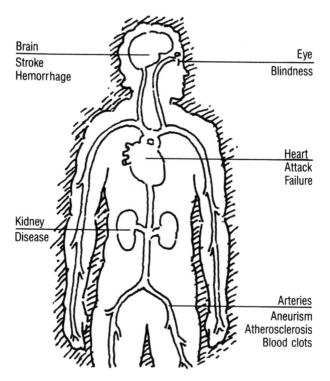

**Figure 7.** Hypertension is a risk factor for developing cardiovascular disease, congestive heart failure, stroke, eye disorders, and kidney disease.

Not everyone who consumes a high-salt diet develops hypertension, which implies that some people might be salt-sensitive.[46]

In recent years, researchers have begun to look at other nutrients for their possible role in hypertension. Studies have shown that dietary calcium has an effect on blood pressure.

## Calcium And Hypertension

The link between calcium intake and risk for hypertension is not new. Observations in the early 1900s showed people who lived in areas with hard water had less heart disease.[47] Hard water contains calcium while soft water has a low calcium and high sodium content. This finding led researchers to study calcium and its effect on blood pressure. Nutritional studies have linked calcium intake to blood pressure levels.[48-51]

The results of these nutrition surveys are interesting. Although the dietary intake of calcium in people with hypertension is lower than in healthy people, the intake is within the "normal" range. If people with hypertension require an increased intake of calcium to prevent or treat hypertension, the RDA might not be sufficient for these people.[52]

Supporting the belief that a low calcium intake also might be associated with hypertension is a study that found two to three times more hypertension among women with osteoporosis than women without this bone disorder.[53]

Not only is a deficiency of calcium linked to hypertension, but when calcium intake is increased, blood pressure often decreases. This effect on blood pressure is seen in healthy people, and people with mild to severe hypertension. The earlier calcium supplementation is started, the greater the long-term effects on lowering blood pressure.[54]

Just how a higher calcium intake might protect against hypertension is not well understood. One theory links calcium in the maintenance of the muscles that surround arteries and help regulate blood pressure.

Another theory states that calcium and magnesium balance at the cellular level might have an effect on blood pressure. Normally, calcium concentration is low within the cell and high outside the cell. Magnesium concentration is the reverse, high within the cell and low outside the cell. This difference in concentrations is maintained by a pumping mechanism in the cell membrane. If the pumping action is defective, these differences in calcium and magnesium concentrations might not be maintained. Too much magnesium might leak out of the cell or too much calcium might leak into the cell. This might disturb the hormone that regulates blood pressure and lead to hypertension.[50,55] If this theory is correct, some people would respond to magnesium supplementation and others would respond to calcium supplementation.[50,55,56]

There might be a link between sodium and calcium intake and hypertension. A diet high in sodium is associated with hypertension and with an increased excretion of calcium.[57] Whether sodium's link with hypertension is independent of calcium or is secondary to an effect on calcium loss has not been determined.

Although the evidence is supportive, the link between calcium and hypertension is not proven. Low blood levels of calcium might be a result of hypertension rather than the cause, in which case an increase in dietary calcium would not benefit the person with elevated blood pressure. However, if low intake of calcium is a cause of hypertension, increased dietary intake or supplementation would be beneficial.

Calcium intake has declined in the United States and is below acceptable levels in some segments of the population such as blacks and older adults; populations that are at high risk for hypertension.[52]

It is too early to make a specific recommendation regarding the amount of calcium a hypertensive person should consume; however, the consumption of a diet that is adequate in calcium, at least 800 mg, would be a beginning. As research progresses, calcium supplementation may emerge as a valuable, inexpensive means of treatment for some people with hypertension.[58] *(Table 3)*

## Other Nutritional Factors And Hypertension

**Calories:** Calorie intake might be the most important dietary factor in the development of hypertension. An increase in weight is associated with an increase in blood pressure.[59] Obese individuals have higher blood

| Table 3 | Calcium Equivalents |
|---|---|
| | The following foods provide the same amount of calcium as an 8 ounce glass of nonfat milk: |
| | **1 cup** calcium-fortified soy milk |
| | **1 cup** broccoli or collards |
| | **1 cup** almonds |
| | **1¼ cups** turnip greens |
| | **1½ cups** kale or mustard greens |
| | **1⅔ cups** sunflower seeds |
| | **2 cups** beet greens |
| | **2 cups** quick-cooking, enriched farina |
| | **3 cups** cooked dried beans |
| | **3 pieces** enriched cornbread |

pressure levels than people who are at their ideal body weight. Weight reduction lowers blood pressure even when sodium intake remains constant.[48]

**Fat:** Some polyunsaturated fats might lower blood pressure by their effect on relaxing the muscles in the artery wall.[59] However, a diet high in fat, especially saturated fats from dairy and animal products, might increase blood pressure.[60]

**Magnesium:** Magnesium is another mineral that might be important in the regulation of blood pressure. Evidence suggests that magnesium may offer as much protection as calcium against hypertension.[50]

**Potassium And Sodium Balance:** Potassium and sodium interact together in the body, and the balance of these two minerals might be a factor in blood pressure. Americans consume more sodium than potassium.[61] High-sodium processed foods, such as potato chips, often replace high-potassium foods, such as fresh fruits and vegetables. This high sodium-low potassium diet might be a factor in hypertension. In some cases, an increase in dietary potassium lowers blood pressure.[62] *(Table 4, Page 45)*

**Chloride:** Table salt is composed of the two elements sodium and chloride. Although sodium is the primary component of salt associated with hypertension, some evidence suggests that chloride also might be involved. Some animals develop hypertension when fed sodium chloride (table salt) but maintain normal blood pressure when fed nonchloride-containing sodium.[59]

**Other Trace Nutrients:** Several trace minerals and vitamins might be involved in the regulation of blood pressure. The trace minerals, including chromium, cobalt, copper, manganese, molybdenum, selenium, vanadium, and zinc, are involved in processes important to cardiovascular health. Several vitamins including vitamin E, vitamin A, vitamin C, and the B vitamins are necessary for the maintenance of cell membranes and other body structures that help regulate blood pressure.[59]

**Summary:** Hypertension is a serious disorder that affects a large portion of the population in the United States. In most cases, the exact cause of hypertension is not known. Various nutritional factors have been implicated in the cause of hypertension. Manipulating the diet, especially to reduce its sodium content, is a popular treatment for hypertension. Calcium has recently emerged as an important nutrient that might prevent hypertension. *(Figure 8)*

**Figure 8. The Antihypertension Diet**

Many questions remain unanswered about calcium and hypertension. As research progresses these questions should be answered. Meanwhile, the safest course of action is for all individuals with hypertension, and those at risk for this disorder, to consume diets that contain at least the recommended daily amount of calcium.

| Table 4 | The Highs And Lows Of Sodium |
|---|---|

**Emphasize These** Foods Low In Sodium
- Unsalted seasonings
- Unsalted grain products
- Baked products made without salt, baking powder or baking soda
- Fruits
- Fruit juices
- Unsalted vegetables
- Fresh meat prepared without salt
- Dried beans cooked without salt or salt pork
- Unsalted nuts
- Ricotta cheese
- Sherbet
- Most mineral waters (check with supplier)

**Use In Moderation** Foods Medium In Sodium
- Lightly salted seasonings
- Tomato puree or sauce
- Grain products made with small amounts of salt, baking powder, or baking soda
- Biscuits and muffins
- Lightly salted vegetables
- Canned vegetables
- Fresh shellfish
- Milk
- Buttermilk
- Yogurt

**Beware of These** Foods High In Sodium
- Salt
- Highly salted seasonings
- Highly salted grain products
- Pretzels
- Salted crackers and chips
- Salted popcorn
- Highly salted vegetables
- All pickled vegetables
- Olives and pickles
- Sauerkraut
- Smoked, cured or pickled products
- Bacon
- Luncheon meats
- American cheese
- Processed cheese products

# 5
# Calcium And Other Health Problems

Calcium might be involved in the treatment and prevention of other diseases and conditions in addition to osteoporosis and hypertension.

## Alzheimer's Disease

An excessive accumulation of aluminum has been observed in the brains of patients with Alzheimer's Disease.[63] Adequate intake of calcium might reduce the toxic effects and accumulation of aluminum in tissues.[64]

## Vitamin D And Bowel Cancer

Calcium and vitamin D might offer some protection against cancer of the colon and rectum. In examining a group of 1,527 men, those men who developed bowel cancer consumed less calcium and vitamin D than those who remained free of this disease.[65] Insufficient evidence exists, however, to recommend an increase in calcium beyond the current RDA to prevent or treat bowel cancer.

## Cardiovascular Disease

Calcium might reduce blood cholesterol levels in some individuals. Elevated blood cholesterol is a risk factor for cardiovascular disease (CVD) and a reduction in blood cholesterol is associated with a reduced risk for CVD. People who have high cholesterol levels sometimes show a reduction in these levels when calcium supplements of 1,000 mg per day are included in the diet.[66]

## Eclampsia Of Pregnancy

Eclampsia is a serious complication of pregnancy that is fatal to the fetus in 30% to 35% of the cases.[67] The disorder is characterized by hypertension, edema (bloating and swelling of the legs or ankles), and protein loss in the urine. Eclampsia, also called toxemia of pregnancy or pre-eclampsia, usually develops in the last three months of pregnancy. The cause of eclampsia is not known but several factors including poor prenatal care, poor nutrition, and first pregnancy are associated with the disease. Low intake of calcium might be related to the development of eclampsia.[68]

A nutritious diet combined with a vitamin-mineral supplement that contains calcium might reduce the incidence of eclampsia.[69]

## Kidney Stones

About 1 in 1,000 adults develops urinary tract stones and is hospitalized as a result of complications.[70] Kidney stones are composed of crystals of calcium combined with other subtances such as oxalate or phosphate. The formation of crystals depends upon the concentration of these substances in the urine; when the concentration is high, stones are more likely to form. Those people who form stones excrete large amounts of calcium, thereby increasing the concentration of calcium in the urine. Calcium supplements are not recommended for individuals prone to developing kidney stones. A physician should be consulted by those people at risk for developing kidney stones, and a diet should be designed that supplies the proper amount of dietary calcium to prevent both osteoporosis and kidney stone formation.

## Periodontal Disease

Diseases of the gums are called periodontal diseases. They are a major cause of tooth loss in adults. Evidence shows that calcium supplementation of 1,000 to 2,000 mg a day over several months might reduce the incidence of periodontal disorders. A diet low in calcium might contribute to the progression of this disease.[71] Inadequate dietary calcium is linked to loss of calcium from the jaw bone (alveolar bone), which makes dentures difficult to position.[39,72] Daily brushing and flossing also are important in the prevention of dental disease.

# 6
# Calcium Supplements

## Who Might Benefit From Calcium Supplementation?

Many people do not consume enough calcium, and calcium supplements are one way for Americans to meet their daily requirements.[3,4]

Women might benefit most from regular calcium supplementation because they consume less calcium and food than men consume. Women also are at higher risk for developing osteoporosis. However, careful consideration of calcium intake is important for all ages, male and female, since anyone can develop osteoporosis.

There are subgroups of people who are at higher risk than others for developing osteoporosis.

- Postmenopausal women,
- People who diet,
- People who are small-boned,
- People who consume several cups of coffee each day,
- People who take medications that reduce calcium absorption, such as tetracycline and aluminum-containing antacids,
- People who smoke cigarettes,
- Women who have had their ovaries surgically removed, and
- People under chronic stress.

## Are All Calcium Supplements Similar?

All calcium supplements are not the same. Calcium is combined with other compounds in supplements. There are five primary types of calcium preparations available. These are:

- Calcium gluconate
- Calcium lactate
- Calcium phosphate
- Calcium carbonate
- Calcium citrate

In healthy individuals, all calcium supplements are absorbed the same and are considered good sources of the mineral. However, some disorders might affect the absorption of different calcium preparations. Calcium requires an acidic environment in the intestine to be absorbed. People with achlorhydria (poor secretion of stomach acid) might not efficiently absorb calcium carbonate. A supplement of calcium citrate, or consuming calcium carbonate with a meal, might improve the absorption of calcium.[73]

Another difference in calcium supplements is the amount of calcium they contain. Calcium carbonate contains the most calcium; it is 40% calcium and 60% carbonate. Calcium phosphate contains 29% calcium. Calcium lactate and calcium gluconate contain between 9% and 13% calcium.[21] People who take calcium must consider this percentage factor when determining how much calcium they are ingesting. *(Table 5, Page 51)*

Some antacid preparations contain large amounts of calcium carbonate and are an excellent source of calcium.[21] One advantage of this type of product is

| Table 5 | The Amount Of Calcium In Different Supplements | | |
|---|---|---|---|
| Calcium Salt | Theoretical Tablet Size | Percent Calcium | Content Of Elemental Calcium |
| Calcium gluconate | 1200 mg | 9 | 108 mg |
| Calcium lactate | 1200 mg | 13 | 156 mg |
| Calcium phosphate | 1200 mg | 29 | 348 mg |
| Calcium carbonate | 1200 mg | 40 | 480 mg |

that the tablets are chewable and often come in a variety of flavors. Use of antacids appears to be a safe practice providing the product does not contain aluminum. Aluminum reduces calcium absorption and encourages the development of bone disorders.[74,75]

Supplements of bone meal and dolomite might be contaminated with trace amounts of toxic metals such as lead, arsenic, mercury, and cadmium.[21] These sources of calcium should be avoided, unless it can be verified that there is no contamination.

Vitamin D is an important regulator of calcium absorption by the body. Before vitamin D can perform its functions in the body, the liver must convert it into an active form. It is this active form that is needed for the absorption of calcium and the regulation of calcium into and out of bone. Older adults might be less efficient at manufacturing vitamin D in the presence of sunlight and at converting vitamin D to its active form.[76] Older adults also might receive less exposure to sunlight and consume fewer foods fortified with vitamin D, making them at higher risk for marginal deficiencies of this nutrient.[35]

Several supplements of calcium contain vitamin D to help boost the body's absorption of calcium. Daily intake of vitamin D should not exceed 800 IU or a level twice the RDA because vitamin D can be toxic at large doses. If selecting a supplement with both calcium and vitamin D, the dosage of each nutrient must be considered.

For people who choose to take calcium supplements or are instructed to do so by their physicians, the amount needed may depend on several factors:

- The amount of calcium consumed in foods. A milk drinker can get approximately 300 mg of calcium in an 8 oz glass. Two glasses of milk a day would almost meet the RDA and require minimal amounts of calcium from a supplement. An individual who is lactose intolerant, dieting, or who dislikes milk might consume far less than 800 mg per day and require more calcium by supplemention.
- Age, gender, physical activity level, and identified risk factors for developing osteoporosis. Premenopausal women or women treated with estrogen should consume 1,000 mg of calcium daily. Postmenopausal women who do not received estrogen treatment should consume 1,500 mg of calcium daily.[26] Achieving these intake levels through diet alone might be difficult.
- Medical conditions or treatments that affect the need for nutrient supplementation. Some conditions may require more calcium and supplements are needed to meet the higher requirements. For others, calcium supplements could be hazardous. A pharmacist should be consulted regarding medication-calcium interactions.

## Are Large Doses Of Calcium Harmful?

Calcium intakes in the range of 1,000 to 2,500 mg daily do not cause problems for normal, healthy individuals.[4]

Information on the effects of large doses of calcium (10,000 mg a day) is limited. If the mineral is hazardous in large amounts it might be because of its effect on the body's balance of other nutrients. Excess intake of calcium might inhibit the absorption of zinc and cause a zinc deficiency. The effect of large doses of calcium on zinc cannot be counteracted with an increased intake of zinc, since large doses of zinc might cause an iron or copper deficiency. Iron absorption and tissue stores might decline when calcium intake is too high.[16]

Large doses of calcium in animals sometimes results in a secondary deficiency of vitamin K and excessive bleeding. Finally, a large intake of calcium might upset the ratio of calcium to phosphorus and result in bone loss.[77]

Calcium supplements can cause minor problems for healthy people. Some people experience constipation, bloating, or intestinal gas.[62] These problems are not serious but can be annoying. Calcium supplements can reduce the effectiveness of tetracycline and should be taken at a different time of the day than the medication.

Calcium supplementation might not be beneficial for people with certain disorders. People with a history of kidney problems should avoid calcium supplementation unless it is specifically prescribed by a physician.

Persons who suffer from peptic ulcer disease may be susceptible to problems from excess calcium intake. A syndrome described as the ''milk-alkalai syndrome" occurs in individuals who consume large amounts of milk along with quantities of antacids. These individuals develop abnormally high levels of calcium in their blood and are more likely to develop kidney problems.[4]

## Summary

The aches and pains, stooped posture, loss of teeth, and bone fractures of osteoporosis and an elevation in blood pressure were once called the inevitable result of "old age." It is now recognized that these diseases are influenced by a lifetime of habits.

The choices a person makes about diet, exercise, and other health habits will have an effect on whether the bones remain strong and upright or become porous and hunched, and whether the blood pressure and heart will remain healthy.

| Worksheet 1 | What Is Your Calcium Intake? | | | |
|---|---|---|---|---|
| **Food** | **Portion Of** | **Number Of Servings** | **Calcium Mg** | **Total Calcium** |
| Plain Lowfat Yogurt | 1 cup | _____ | | |
| Nonfat Dry Milk Powder | 1/2 cup | _____ | | |
| Canned Sardines (with bones) | 3 oz. | + _____ | | |
| | *Total Servings* | _____ | × 400 = | _____ |
| Fruit Flavored Yogurt | 1 cup | _____ | | |
| Skim and Lowfat Milk | 1 cup | _____ | | |
| Whole Milk, Buttermilk, Choc. Milk | 1 cup | _____ | | |
| Parmesan Cheese (grated) | 1/4 cup | _____ | | |
| Swiss and Gruyere Cheese | 1 oz. | + _____ | | |
| | *Total Servings* | _____ | × 300 = | _____ |
| Cheese (all other hard cheese) | 1 oz. | _____ | | |
| Enriched Farina (instant, cooked) | 1 cup | + _____ | | |
| | *Total Servings* | _____ | × 200 = | _____ |
| Canned Pink Salmon (with bones) | 3 oz. | _____ | | |
| Collards and Turnip Greens, cooked | 1/2 cup | _____ | | |
| Tofu (processed with calcium) | 4 oz. | + _____ | | |
| | *Total Servings* | _____ | × 150 = | _____ |

*(Continued on next page)*

| Food | Portion Of | Number Of Servings | Calcium Mg | Total Calcium |
|------|-----------|-------------------|-----------|---------------|
| Ice Cream and Ice Milk | 1/2 cup | | | |
| Spinach, cooked | 1/2 cup | _____ | | |
| Broccoli, cooked | 1/2 cup | + _____ | | |
| | *Total Servings* | _____ | × 75 = | _____ |
| Almonds | 1 oz. | _____ | | |
| Soybeans, cooked | 1/2 cup | _____ | | |
| Chard, cooked | 1/2 cup | _____ | | |
| Cottage Cheese | 1/2 cup | _____ | | |
| Corn Tortilla | 1 med. | _____ | | |
| Orange | 1 med | _____ | | |
| Kidney, Lima and Navy Beans, cooked | 1/2 cup | + _____ | | |
| | *Total Servings* | _____ | × 50 = | _____ |
| Carrot, raw | 1 med | _____ | | |
| Dates and Raisins | 1/4 cup | _____ | | |
| Egg | 1 large | _____ | | |
| Whole Wheat Bread | 1 slice | _____ | | |
| Peanut Butter | 2 Tbsp | + _____ | | |
| | *Total Servings* | _____ | × 25 = | _____ |

My Actual Calcium Intake ........................ _____

Less My RDA For Calcium ..................... _____

The Difference Is ............................. _____

# References

1. *Recommended Dietary Allowances,* 9 ed, 1980. National Academy of Sciences, Washington, DC, pp 125-132.
2. Recker R: Osteoporosis. *Cont Nutr* 1983; 8:1-2
3. Garrison R, Somer E: *The Nutrition Desk Reference.* New Canaan, Conn, Keats Publishing Co 1985, pp 116-124.
4. Heaney R, Gallagher J, Johnston C, et al: Calcium nutrition and bone health in the elderly. *Am J Clin Nutr* 1982; 36:986-1013.
5. Keyler D, Peterson C: Oral calcium supplements: How much or what, for whom, and why? *Postgr Med* 1985; 78:123-125.
6. Chinn H: Effects of dietary factors on skeletal integrity in adults. *Calcium, Phosphorus, Vitamin D and Protein.* Report for FDA Contract 223-79-2775, Bethesda MD: Life Science Reseach Office FASEB, 1981.
7. Brewster L, Jacobson M: *The Changing American Diet: A Chronicle of American Eating Habits From 1910-1980.* Washington DC, Center For Science in the Public Interest. 1983, p 74.
8. Pao E, Mickle S: Problem nutrients in the United States. *Food Tech* 1981; 35:58-69.
9. Brewster L, Jacobson M: *The Changing American Diet: A Chronical of American Eating Habits From 1910-1980.* Washington DC, Center For Science in the Public Interest. 1983, p 39.
10. Newcomer A, Hodgson S, McGill D, et al: Lactase deficiency: Prevalence in osteoporosis. *Ann Int Med* 1978; 89:218-220.
11. Goodhart R, Shils M: *Modern Nutrition in Health and Disease,* 6th Ed. Philadelphia, Lea & Febiger, 1980, pp 295-309.
12. Czajka-Narins D: Minerals, in Krause M, Mahan L (eds): *Food, Nutrition, and Diet Therapy,* ed 7. Philadelphia, WB Saunders Co, 1984, pp 150-151.
13. Gallagher J, Jerpbak C, Gee W, et al: 1,25 dihydroxy-vitamin D3:Short- and long-term effects on bone and calcium metabolism in patients with postmenopausal osteoporosis. *Proc Natl Acad Sci* 1982; 79:3325.

14. Wills M: Intestinal absorption of calcium. *Lancet* 1973; 1:820.
15. Taylor A, Wasserman R: Vitamin D-induced calcium binding protein: Comparative aspects in kidney and intestine. *Am J Physiol* 1972; 223:110.
16. Marcus R: Calcium, skeletal aging, and osteoporosis. *Nutr & MD* 1985; 11:1-6.
17. Song M, Adham N, Ament M: A possible role of zinc on the intestinal calcium absorption mechanisms. *Nutr Rep Int* 1985; 31:43-51.
18. Carroll M, Abraham S, Dresser C: *Dietary Intake Source Data: United States, 1976-1980.* US Dept Health and Human Services Publ No. (HS) 83-1681. Washington, DC, US Government Printing Office, 1983.
19. Dairy Council Digest: Calcium: Utilization and Requirement, in Labuza T, Sloan A: *Contemporary Nutrition Controversies.* St Paul, West Publishing Co, 1979, pp 202-210.
20. Heaney R: *Prevention of Age-related Osteoporosis in Women, The Osteoporotic Sydrome,* New York, Grune & Stratton 1983, pp 123-144.
21. Fanelli M: Promoting women's health. *Dietetic Currents* 1985; 12-4:19-24.
22. Davies R, Saha S: Osteoporosis. *Am Fam Phys* 1985; 32:107-114.
23. Are you at risk for bone disease? Rosemont, Illinois, *National Dairy Council* 1984, 60018-4233.
24. Riggs B: Changes in bone mineral density of the proximal femur and spine with aging. *J Clin Invest* 1982; 70:716.
25. Guyton A: *Textbook of Medical Physiology,* ed 5. Philadelphia, WB Saunders Co 1976, pp 1056-1059.
26. Osteoporosis-Consensus Conference: *JAMA* 1984; 252:799-802.
27. Albanese A: Problems of bone health in elderly. *NY State J Med* 1975; 75:326.
28. Osteoporosis and calcium balance. *Nutrition Reviews* 1983; 41:83-85.
29. Lane J, Vigorita V: Osteoporosis. *J Bone Joint Surg* 1983; 65-A:274-278.

30. Marcus R: The relationship of dietary calcium to the maintenance of skeletal integrity in man. *Metabolism* 1982; 31:93.
31. Mack R, La Chance P: Effects of recumbancy and space flight on bone density. *Am J Clin Nutr* 1967; 20:1194.
32. Keyler D, Peterson D: Oral calcium supplements: How much of what, for whom and why? *Postgrad Med* 1985; 78:123-125.
33. Spencer, H, Kramer L, Norris C, et al: Effect of small doses of aluminum-containing antacids on calcium and phosphorus metabolism. *Am J Clin Nutr* 1982; 36:776.
34. Recker R: Osteoporosis. *Cont Nutr* 1983; 8:1-2.
35. MacLaughlin J, Holick M: Aging decreases the capacity of human skin to produce vitamin D3. *J Clin Inv* 1985; 76:1536-1538.
36. Fluoride and osteoporosis. *Nutr & MD* 1979; 5:5.
37. Albanese A: Calcium nutrition in the elderly. *Nutr & MD* 1979; V:1-6.
38. Ludwack L: Dietary calcium and reversal of bone mineralization. Rosemont, Illinois, *Nutr News* 1974; 37:1.
39. Krook L: Experimental studies on osteoporosis, in Jasmin D, Cantin M (eds): *Methods and Achievements in Experimental Pathology.* Montreal, Karger, Basel 1975; 7:72.
40. The 1984 Report of the Joint National Committee on Detection, Evaluation, and Treatment of High Blood Pressure. *Arch Int Med* 1984; 144:1045-1057.
41. Symposium: Hypertension and Antihypertensive drugs. *Fed Proc* 1981; 40:2250.
42. Rowland F, Roberts J: *Blood Pressure Levels in Persons 6-74 Years: United States 1976-1980,* Advance data. National Center for Health Statistics, Vital and Health Statistics No. 84. US Dept of Health and Human Services, Public Health Service, Oct, 1982.
43. Garrison R, Somer E: *The Nutrition Desk Reference.* New Canaan, Conn, Keats Publishing Co, 1985, p 155.
44. Dahl K: Salt and hypertension. *Am J Clin Nutr* 1972; 25:231.

45. Tobian L.: Dietary salt (sodium) and hypertension. *Am J Clin Nutr* 1979; 32:2659-2662.

46. MacGregor G: Double-blind, randomized cross-over trial of moderate sodium restriction in essential hypertension. *Lancet* 1982; 1:351-354.

47. Schroeder H: Relation between mortality for cardiovascular disease and treated water supplies. *JAMA* 1960; 172: 1902-1908.

48. McCarron D, Henry H, Morris C: Human nutrition and blood pressure regulation: an integrated approach. *Hypertension* 1982; 4(suppIII):III2-III3.

49. Ackley S, Barrett-Connor E, Suarez L: Dairy products, calcium, and blood pressure. *Am J Clin Nutr* 1983; 38:457-461.

50. McCarron D: Calcium and magnesium nutrition in human hypertension. *Ann Int Med* 1983; 98:800-805.

51. Belizan J, Villar J, Pineda O, et al: Reduction of blood pressure with calcium supplementation in young adults. *JAMA* 1983; 249:1161.

52. McCarron D, Morris C, Cole C: Dietary calcium in human hypertension. *Science* 1982; 217:267-269.

53. McCarron D, Chestnut C, Baylink, D: Blood pressure response to the pharmacological management of osteoporosis. *Clin Res* 1981; 29:274A.

54. McCarron D: Proceedings of the 4th International Symposium on rats with spontaneous hypertension. Schattauel, Stuttgart 1982, p 421.

55. Resnick L: Divalent cations in essential hypertension — relations between serum ionized calcium magnesium and plasma renin activity. *N Eng J Med* 1983; 309:888-891.

56. Cranton E: Calcium: The two-edged sword. *Corporate Fitness and Recreation* 1983; Aug-Sept:13-14.

57. Dietary factors and blood pressure. *Dairy Council Digest* 1981; 52:25-30.

58. Resnick L: Calcium and hypertension: The emerging connection. *Ann of Int Med* 1985; 103:944-945.

59. Henry H, McCarron D: Diet and hypertension: An update on recent research. *Cont Nutr* 1982; 7:1-2.

60. Puska P, Iacono J, Nissinen A, et al: Dietary fat and blood pressure: An intervention study on the effects of

a low-fat diet with two levels of polyunsaturated fat. *Prev Med* 1985; 14:573-584.

61. Shank F, Park Y, Harland B, et al: Perspective of food and drug administration on dietary sodium. *J Am Diet Assoc* 1982; 80:29-35.

62. MacGregor G, Smith S, Markandu M, et al: Moderate potassium supplementation and essential hypertension. *Lancet* 1982; 2:567.

63. Koning J: Aluminum pots as a source of dietary aluminum. *N Eng J Med* 1981; 304:172.

64. Garrison R, Somer E: *The Nutrition Desk Reference.* New Canaan, Conn, Keats Publishing Co 1985, p 106.

65. Calcium and vitamin D intakes influence the risk of bowel cancer in men. *Nutr Rev* 1985; 43:170

66. Karanja N: Dietary and serum lipid levels in humans: response to oral calcium. *Fed Proc* 1985; 44:817.

67. Villar J: Epidemiological observations on the relationship between calcium intake and eclampsia. *Int J Gyn Obst* 1983; 21:271.

68. Belizan J, Villar J: The relationship between calcium intake and edema-, proteinuria-, and hypertension-gestosis: an hypothesis. *Am J Clin Nutr* 1980; 33:2202-2210.

69. Worthington-Roberts B: Nutrition during pregnancy and lactation, in Krause M, Mahan L: *Food, Nutrition, and Diet Therapy,* ed 7. Philadelphia, WB Saunders Co 1984, p 261.

70. Magnesium: Protector Against Kidney Stones. *The Supplement* 1984; 4(5):1.

71. Rottka H, Pieper R, von Herrath D, et al: The influence of the calcium/phosphorus ratio in the diet on human bone disease, the role of nutritive secondary hyperparathyroidism. *Int J Vit Nutr Res* 1981; 51:373-379.

72. Krause M, Mahan L: *Food, Nutrition, and Diet Therapy,* ed 7. Philadelphia, WB Saunders Co 1984, p 687.

73. Recker R: Calcium absorption and achlorhydria. *N Eng J Med* 1985; 31:70-73.

74. Robertson J, Felsenfeld A, Haygood C, et al: Animal model of aluminum induced osteomalacia: Role of chronic renal failure. *Kidney Int* 1983; 23:327-335.

75. Goodman W, Gilligan J, Horst R: Short term aluminum adminstration in the rat. *J Clin Inv* 1984; 73:171-181.
76. Tsai K, Heath H, Kumar R, et al: Impaired vitamin D metabolism with aging in women. *J Clin Invest* 1984; 73:166.
77. Calcium: How much is too much? *Nutr Rev* 1985; 43:345-346.

## Glossary

**Alveolar Bone:** The jaw bone.

**Artery:** Blood vessel that carries blood and oxygen from the heart to the tissues.

**Bacteria:** Microscopic one-celled organisms found in food and in the body.

**Caffeine:** A drug that stimulates the nervous system and is found in coffee, tea, and some soft drinks.

**Calorie:** A measurement of heat. In nutrition, calorie refers to the quantity of energy contained in foods.

**Cardiovascular Disease:** A disease of the heart and blood vessels often caused by an accumulation of cholesterol in the lining of the blood vessels.

**Cholesterol:** A type of fat found in foods from animal sources and also produced by the liver. High levels of cholesterol in the blood are associated with the development of cardiovascular disease.

**Collagen:** A protein found in connective tissue, bone, skin, and tendons that holds cells and other substances together.

**Cortical Bone:** A type of bone found in the long bones of the arms and legs, characterized by a dense, compacted appearance.

**Dowager's Hump:** The hunched appearance common in people with osteoporosis. The chest also might be collapsed and the abdomen protruded.

**Eclampsia:** A disorder that occurs in the latter three months of pregnancy, characterized by fluid retention, hypertension, protein loss in the urine, convulsions, or coma.

**Enzyme:** Protein-like substances in the body that initiate and accelerate chemical reactions.

**Estrogen:** The female sex hormone that aids in the regulation of ovulation and sex characteristics.

**Hormone:** A chemical substance produced by the endocrine glands that is released into the blood and transported to another organ or tissue, where it performs a specific action. Examples of hormones are estrogen, adrenalin, and insulin.

**Hypertension:** High blood pressure.

**Lactation:** Breastfeeding.

**Lactose:** Milk sugar.

**Lactose Intolerance:** Inability to digest milk sugar (lactose) because of a deficit of lactase, the enzyme that digests lactose.

**Metabolism:** The total of all body processes that converts foods into tissues, breaks down and repairs tissues, and converts complex substances into simple ones for energy.

**Obesity:** Body weight more than 20% above desirable weight; excessive body fat.

**Osteoporosis:** Loss of calcium from the bones that results in porous, weak bones that are prone to fractures.

**Oxalate:** A substance in foods, such as spinach and chard, that binds with calcium and reduces the absorption of the mineral.

**Periodontal Disease:** Diseases of the tissues that surround the teeth.

**Polyunsaturated Fat:** The type of fat found in vegetable oils, nuts, and seeds, and in smaller amounts in fish and chicken.

**Phytate:** A compound found in unleavened whole grain cereals that binds to calcium in the intestine and reduces its absorption.

**Recommended Dietary Allowance (RDA):** The amounts of nutrients recommended by the Food and Nutrition Board of the National Academy of Sciences to meet the needs of most healthy groups of people in the United States.

**Resorption:** Removal of calcium from bone by dissolving into the blood.

**Sodium:** A mineral found in table salt and foods, which is linked to hypertension.

**Tetany:** Intermittent and painful spasms of the muscles.

**Trabecular bone:** A type of bone that is found in the spine and pelvis, characterized by a honeycomb appearance.

**Vertebrae:** Any one of the 33 bones in the spinal column.

# Index

69

# Notes

# Notes

# Notes